DATE

SYMPTOMS

cramping	muscle pain	seizures
anxiety	nerve pain	headache
fatigue	joint pain	dizziness
depression	nausea	eye pressure
appetite loss	stress	spasms

other _____

product used _____

dosage _____

method _____

other meds _____

NOTES

Did your symptoms improve, stay the same, or get worse?

DATE

SYMPTOMS

cramping	muscle pain	seizures
anxiety	nerve pain	headache
fatigue	joint pain	dizziness
depression	nausea	eye pressure
appetite loss	stress	spasms

other _____

product used _____

dosage _____

method _____

other meds _____

NOTES

Did your symptoms improve, stay the same, or get worse?

DATE

SYMPTOMS

cramping	muscle pain	seizures
anxiety	nerve pain	headache
fatigue	joint pain	dizziness
depression	nausea	eye pressure
appetite loss	stress	spasms

other _____

product used _____

dosage _____

method _____

other meds _____

NOTES

Did your symptoms improve, stay the same, or get worse?

DATE

SYMPTOMS

cramping	muscle pain	seizures
anxiety	nerve pain	headache
fatigue	joint pain	dizziness
depression	nausea	eye pressure
appetite loss	stress	spasms

other _____

product used _____

dosage _____

method _____

other meds _____

NOTES

Did your symptoms improve, stay the same, or get worse?

DATE

SYMPTOMS

cramping	muscle pain	seizures
anxiety	nerve pain	headache
fatigue	joint pain	dizziness
depression	nausea	eye pressure
appetite loss	stress	spasms

other _____

product used _____

dosage _____

method _____

other meds _____

NOTES

Did your symptoms improve, stay the same, or get worse?

DATE

SYMPTOMS

cramping	muscle pain	seizures
anxiety	nerve pain	headache
fatigue	joint pain	dizziness
depression	nausea	eye pressure
appetite loss	stress	spasms

other _____

product used _____

dosage _____

method _____

other meds _____

NOTES

Did your symptoms improve, stay the same, or get worse?

DATE

SYMPTOMS

cramping	muscle pain	seizures
anxiety	nerve pain	headache
fatigue	joint pain	dizziness
depression	nausea	eye pressure
appetite loss	stress	spasms

other _____

product used _____

dosage _____

method _____

other meds _____

NOTES

Did your symptoms improve, stay the same, or get worse?

DATE

SYMPTOMS

cramping	muscle pain	seizures
anxiety	nerve pain	headache
fatigue	joint pain	dizziness
depression	nausea	eye pressure
appetite loss	stress	spasms

other _____

product used _____

dosage _____

method _____

other meds _____

NOTES

Did your symptoms improve, stay the same, or get worse?

DATE

SYMPTOMS

cramping	muscle pain	seizures
anxiety	nerve pain	headache
fatigue	joint pain	dizziness
depression	nausea	eye pressure
appetite loss	stress	spasms

other _____

product used _____

dosage _____

method _____

other meds _____

NOTES

Did your symptoms improve, stay the same, or get worse?

DATE

SYMPTOMS

cramping	muscle pain	seizures
anxiety	nerve pain	headache
fatigue	joint pain	dizziness
depression	nausea	eye pressure
appetite loss	stress	spasms

other _____

product used _____

dosage _____

method _____

other meds _____

NOTES

_____

Did your symptoms improve, stay the same, or get worse?

DATE

SYMPTOMS

cramping	muscle pain	seizures
anxiety	nerve pain	headache
fatigue	joint pain	dizziness
depression	nausea	eye pressure
appetite loss	stress	spasms

other _____

product used _____

dosage _____

method _____

other meds _____

NOTES

Did your symptoms improve, stay the same, or get worse?

DATE

SYMPTOMS

cramping	muscle pain	seizures
anxiety	nerve pain	headache
fatigue	joint pain	dizziness
depression	nausea	eye pressure
appetite loss	stress	spasms

other _____

product used _____

dosage _____

method _____

other meds _____

NOTES

Did your symptoms improve, stay the same, or get worse?

DATE

SYMPTOMS

cramping	muscle pain	seizures
anxiety	nerve pain	headache
fatigue	joint pain	dizziness
depression	nausea	eye pressure
appetite loss	stress	spasms

other _____

product used _____

dosage _____

method _____

other meds _____

NOTES

Did your symptoms improve, stay the same, or get worse?

DATE

SYMPTOMS

cramping	muscle pain	seizures
anxiety	nerve pain	headache
fatigue	joint pain	dizziness
depression	nausea	eye pressure
appetite loss	stress	spasms

other _____

product used _____

dosage _____

method _____

other meds _____

NOTES

Did your symptoms improve, stay the same, or get worse?

DATE

SYMPTOMS

cramping	muscle pain	seizures
anxiety	nerve pain	headache
fatigue	joint pain	dizziness
depression	nausea	eye pressure
appetite loss	stress	spasms

other _____

product used _____

dosage _____

method _____

other meds _____

NOTES

Did your symptoms improve, stay the same, or get worse?

DATE

SYMPTOMS

cramping	muscle pain	seizures
anxiety	nerve pain	headache
fatigue	joint pain	dizziness
depression	nausea	eye pressure
appetite loss	stress	spasms

other _____

product used _____

dosage _____

method _____

other meds _____

NOTES

Did your symptoms improve, stay the same, or get worse?

DATE

SYMPTOMS

cramping	muscle pain	seizures
anxiety	nerve pain	headache
fatigue	joint pain	dizziness
depression	nausea	eye pressure
appetite loss	stress	spasms

other _____

product used _____

dosage _____

method _____

other meds _____

NOTES

Did your symptoms improve, stay the same, or get worse?

DATE

SYMPTOMS

cramping	muscle pain	seizures
anxiety	nerve pain	headache
fatigue	joint pain	dizziness
depression	nausea	eye pressure
appetite loss	stress	spasms

other _____

product used _____

dosage _____

method _____

other meds _____

NOTES

Did your symptoms improve, stay the same, or get worse?

DATE

SYMPTOMS

cramping	muscle pain	seizures
anxiety	nerve pain	headache
fatigue	joint pain	dizziness
depression	nausea	eye pressure
appetite loss	stress	spasms

other _____

product used _____

dosage _____

method _____

other meds _____

NOTES

Did your symptoms improve, stay the same, or get worse?

DATE

SYMPTOMS

cramping	muscle pain	seizures
anxiety	nerve pain	headache
fatigue	joint pain	dizziness
depression	nausea	eye pressure
appetite loss	stress	spasms

other _____

product used _____

dosage _____

method _____

other meds _____

NOTES

Did your symptoms improve, stay the same, or get worse?

DATE

SYMPTOMS

cramping	muscle pain	seizures
anxiety	nerve pain	headache
fatigue	joint pain	dizziness
depression	nausea	eye pressure
appetite loss	stress	spasms

other _____

product used _____

dosage _____

method _____

other meds _____

NOTES

Did your symptoms improve, stay the same, or get worse?

DATE

SYMPTOMS

cramping	muscle pain	seizures
anxiety	nerve pain	headache
fatigue	joint pain	dizziness
depression	nausea	eye pressure
appetite loss	stress	spasms

other _____

product used _____

dosage _____

method _____

other meds _____

NOTES

Did your symptoms improve, stay the same, or get worse?

DATE

SYMPTOMS

cramping	muscle pain	seizures
anxiety	nerve pain	headache
fatigue	joint pain	dizziness
depression	nausea	eye pressure
appetite loss	stress	spasms

other _____

product used _____

dosage _____

method _____

other meds _____

NOTES

Did your symptoms improve, stay the same, or get worse?

DATE

SYMPTOMS

cramping   muscle pain   seizures

anxiety   nerve pain   headache

fatigue   joint pain   dizziness

depression   nausea   eye pressure

appetite loss   stress   spasms

other _____

product used _____

dosage _____

method _____

other meds _____

NOTES

Did your symptoms improve, stay the same, or get worse?

DATE

SYMPTOMS

cramping	muscle pain	seizures
anxiety	nerve pain	headache
fatigue	joint pain	dizziness
depression	nausea	eye pressure
appetite loss	stress	spasms

other _____

product used _____

dosage _____

method _____

other meds _____

NOTES

Did your symptoms improve, stay the same, or get worse?

DATE

SYMPTOMS

cramping	muscle pain	seizures
anxiety	nerve pain	headache
fatigue	joint pain	dizziness
depression	nausea	eye pressure
appetite loss	stress	spasms

other _____

product used _____

dosage _____

method _____

other meds _____

NOTES

Did your symptoms improve, stay the same, or get worse?

DATE

SYMPTOMS

cramping	muscle pain	seizures
anxiety	nerve pain	headache
fatigue	joint pain	dizziness
depression	nausea	eye pressure
appetite loss	stress	spasms

other _____

product used _____

dosage _____

method _____

other meds _____

NOTES

Did your symptoms improve, stay the same, or get worse?

DATE

cramping   muscle pain   seizures

anxiety   nerve pain   headache

fatigue   joint pain   dizziness

depression   nausea   eye pressure

appetite loss   stress   spasms

other _____

product used _____

dosage _____

method _____

other meds _____

NOTES

Did your symptoms improve, stay the same, or get worse?

DATE

SYMPTOMS

cramping	muscle pain	seizures
anxiety	nerve pain	headache
fatigue	joint pain	dizziness
depression	nausea	eye pressure
appetite loss	stress	spasms

other _____

product used _____

dosage _____

method _____

other meds _____

NOTES

Did your symptoms improve, stay the same, or get worse?

DATE

SYMPTOMS

cramping	muscle pain	seizures
anxiety	nerve pain	headache
fatigue	joint pain	dizziness
depression	nausea	eye pressure
appetite loss	stress	spasms

other _____

product used _____

dosage _____

method _____

other meds _____

NOTES

Did your symptoms improve, stay the same, or get worse?

DATE

SYMPTOMS

cramping	muscle pain	seizures
anxiety	nerve pain	headache
fatigue	joint pain	dizziness
depression	nausea	eye pressure
appetite loss	stress	spasms

other _____

product used _____

dosage _____

method _____

other meds _____

NOTES

Did your symptoms improve, stay the same, or get worse?

DATE

SYMPTOMS

cramping	muscle pain	seizures
anxiety	nerve pain	headache
fatigue	joint pain	dizziness
depression	nausea	eye pressure
appetite loss	stress	spasms

other _____

product used _____

dosage _____

method _____

other meds _____

NOTES

Did your symptoms improve, stay the same, or get worse?

DATE

SYMPTOMS

cramping	muscle pain	seizures
anxiety	nerve pain	headache
fatigue	joint pain	dizziness
depression	nausea	eye pressure
appetite loss	stress	spasms

other _____

product used _____

dosage _____

method _____

other meds _____

NOTES

Did your symptoms improve, stay the same, or get worse?

DATE

SYMPTOMS

cramping	muscle pain	seizures
anxiety	nerve pain	headache
fatigue	joint pain	dizziness
depression	nausea	eye pressure
appetite loss	stress	spasms

other _____

product used _____

dosage _____

method _____

other meds _____

NOTES

Did your symptoms improve, stay the same, or get worse?

DATE

SYMPTOMS

cramping	muscle pain	seizures
anxiety	nerve pain	headache
fatigue	joint pain	dizziness
depression	nausea	eye pressure
appetite loss	stress	spasms

other _____

product used _____

dosage _____

method _____

other meds _____

NOTES

Did your symptoms improve, stay the same, or get worse?

DATE

SYMPTOMS

cramping	muscle pain	seizures
anxiety	nerve pain	headache
fatigue	joint pain	dizziness
depression	nausea	eye pressure
appetite loss	stress	spasms

other _____

product used _____

dosage _____

method _____

other meds _____

NOTES

Did your symptoms improve, stay the same, or get worse?

DATE

SYMPTOMS

cramping	muscle pain	seizures
anxiety	nerve pain	headache
fatigue	joint pain	dizziness
depression	nausea	eye pressure
appetite loss	stress	spasms

other _____

product used _____

dosage _____

method _____

other meds _____

NOTES

Did your symptoms improve, stay the same, or get worse?

DATE

SYMPTOMS

cramping	muscle pain	seizures
anxiety	nerve pain	headache
fatigue	joint pain	dizziness
depression	nausea	eye pressure
appetite loss	stress	spasms

other _____

product used _____

dosage _____

method _____

other meds _____

NOTES

Did your symptoms improve, stay the same, or get worse?

DATE

SYMPTOMS

cramping	muscle pain	seizures
anxiety	nerve pain	headache
fatigue	joint pain	dizziness
depression	nausea	eye pressure
appetite loss	stress	spasms

other _____

product used _____

dosage _____

method _____

other meds _____

NOTES

Did your symptoms improve, stay the same, or get worse?

DATE

SYMPTOMS

cramping	muscle pain	seizures
anxiety	nerve pain	headache
fatigue	joint pain	dizziness
depression	nausea	eye pressure
appetite loss	stress	spasms

other _____

product used _____

dosage _____

method _____

other meds _____

NOTES

Did your symptoms improve, stay the same, or get worse?

DATE

SYMPTOMS

cramping	muscle pain	seizures
anxiety	nerve pain	headache
fatigue	joint pain	dizziness
depression	nausea	eye pressure
appetite loss	stress	spasms

other _____

product used _____

dosage _____

method _____

other meds _____

NOTES

Did your symptoms improve, stay the same, or get worse?

DATE

SYMPTOMS

cramping	muscle pain	seizures
anxiety	nerve pain	headache
fatigue	joint pain	dizziness
depression	nausea	eye pressure
appetite loss	stress	spasms

other _____

product used _____

dosage _____

method _____

other meds _____

NOTES

Did your symptoms improve, stay the same, or get worse?

DATE

SYMPTOMS

cramping	muscle pain	seizures
anxiety	nerve pain	headache
fatigue	joint pain	dizziness
depression	nausea	eye pressure
appetite loss	stress	spasms

other _____

product used _____

dosage _____

method _____

other meds _____

NOTES

Did your symptoms improve, stay the same, or get worse?

DATE

SYMPTOMS

cramping	muscle pain	seizures
anxiety	nerve pain	headache
fatigue	joint pain	dizziness
depression	nausea	eye pressure
appetite loss	stress	spasms

other _____

product used _____

dosage _____

method _____

other meds _____

NOTES

Did your symptoms improve, stay the same, or get worse?

DATE

SYMPTOMS

cramping	muscle pain	seizures
anxiety	nerve pain	headache
fatigue	joint pain	dizziness
depression	nausea	eye pressure
appetite loss	stress	spasms

other _____

product used _____

dosage _____

method _____

other meds _____

NOTES

Did your symptoms improve, stay the same, or get worse?

DATE

SYMPTOMS

cramping	muscle pain	seizures
anxiety	nerve pain	headache
fatigue	joint pain	dizziness
depression	nausea	eye pressure
appetite loss	stress	spasms

other _____

product used _____

dosage _____

method _____

other meds _____

NOTES

Did your symptoms improve, stay the same, or get worse?

DATE

SYMPTOMS

cramping	muscle pain	seizures
anxiety	nerve pain	headache
fatigue	joint pain	dizziness
depression	nausea	eye pressure
appetite loss	stress	spasms

other _____

product used _____

dosage _____

method _____

other meds _____

NOTES

Did your symptoms improve, stay the same, or get worse?

DATE

SYMPTOMS

cramping	muscle pain	seizures
anxiety	nerve pain	headache
fatigue	joint pain	dizziness
depression	nausea	eye pressure
appetite loss	stress	spasms

other _____

product used _____

dosage _____

method _____

other meds _____

NOTES

Did your symptoms improve, stay the same, or get worse?

DATE

SYMPTOMS

cramping	muscle pain	seizures
anxiety	nerve pain	headache
fatigue	joint pain	dizziness
depression	nausea	eye pressure
appetite loss	stress	spasms

other _____

product used _____

dosage _____

method _____

other meds _____

NOTES

Did your symptoms improve, stay the same, or get worse?

DATE

SYMPTOMS

cramping	muscle pain	seizures
anxiety	nerve pain	headache
fatigue	joint pain	dizziness
depression	nausea	eye pressure
appetite loss	stress	spasms

other _____

product used _____

dosage _____

method _____

other meds _____

NOTES

Did your symptoms improve, stay the same, or get worse?

DATE

SYMPTOMS

cramping	muscle pain	seizures
anxiety	nerve pain	headache
fatigue	joint pain	dizziness
depression	nausea	eye pressure
appetite loss	stress	spasms

other _____

product used _____

dosage _____

method _____

other meds _____

NOTES

Did your symptoms improve, stay the same, or get worse?

DATE

SYMPTOMS

cramping	muscle pain	seizures
anxiety	nerve pain	headache
fatigue	joint pain	dizziness
depression	nausea	eye pressure
appetite loss	stress	spasms

other _____

product used _____

dosage _____

method _____

other meds _____

NOTES

Did your symptoms improve, stay the same, or get worse?

DATE

SYMPTOMS

cramping	muscle pain	seizures
anxiety	nerve pain	headache
fatigue	joint pain	dizziness
depression	nausea	eye pressure
appetite loss	stress	spasms

other _____

product used _____

dosage _____

method _____

other meds _____

NOTES

Did your symptoms improve, stay the same, or get worse?

DATE

SYMPTOMS

cramping	muscle pain	seizures
anxiety	nerve pain	headache
fatigue	joint pain	dizziness
depression	nausea	eye pressure
appetite loss	stress	spasms

other _____

product used _____

dosage _____

method _____

other meds _____

NOTES

Did your symptoms improve, stay the same, or get worse?

DATE

SYMPTOMS

cramping	muscle pain	seizures
anxiety	nerve pain	headache
fatigue	joint pain	dizziness
depression	nausea	eye pressure
appetite loss	stress	spasms

other _____

product used _____

dosage _____

method _____

other meds _____

NOTES

Did your symptoms improve, stay the same, or get worse?

DATE

SYMPTOMS

cramping	muscle pain	seizures
anxiety	nerve pain	headache
fatigue	joint pain	dizziness
depression	nausea	eye pressure
appetite loss	stress	spasms

other _____

product used _____

dosage _____

method _____

other meds _____

NOTES

Did your symptoms improve, stay the same, or get worse?

DATE

SYMPTOMS

cramping	muscle pain	seizures
anxiety	nerve pain	headache
fatigue	joint pain	dizziness
depression	nausea	eye pressure
appetite loss	stress	spasms

other _____

product used _____

dosage _____

method _____

other meds _____

NOTES

Did your symptoms improve, stay the same, or get worse?

DATE

SYMPTOMS

cramping	muscle pain	seizures
anxiety	nerve pain	headache
fatigue	joint pain	dizziness
depression	nausea	eye pressure
appetite loss	stress	spasms

other _____

product used _____

dosage _____

method _____

other meds _____

NOTES

Did your symptoms improve, stay the same, or get worse?

DATE

SYMPTOMS

cramping	muscle pain	seizures
anxiety	nerve pain	headache
fatigue	joint pain	dizziness
depression	nausea	eye pressure
appetite loss	stress	spasms

other _____

product used _____

dosage _____

method _____

other meds _____

NOTES

Did your symptoms improve, stay the same, or get worse?

DATE

cramping	muscle pain	seizures
anxiety	nerve pain	headache
fatigue	joint pain	dizziness
depression	nausea	eye pressure
appetite loss	stress	spasms

other _____

product used _____

dosage _____

method _____

other meds _____

NOTES

Did your symptoms improve, stay the same, or get worse?

DATE

SYMPTOMS

cramping	muscle pain	seizures
anxiety	nerve pain	headache
fatigue	joint pain	dizziness
depression	nausea	eye pressure
appetite loss	stress	spasms

other _____

product used _____

dosage _____

method _____

other meds _____

NOTES

Did your symptoms improve, stay the same, or get worse?

DATE

SYMPTOMS

cramping	muscle pain	seizures
anxiety	nerve pain	headache
fatigue	joint pain	dizziness
depression	nausea	eye pressure
appetite loss	stress	spasms

other _____

product used _____

dosage _____

method _____

other meds _____

NOTES

Did your symptoms improve, stay the same, or get worse?

DATE

SYMPTOMS

cramping	muscle pain	seizures
anxiety	nerve pain	headache
fatigue	joint pain	dizziness
depression	nausea	eye pressure
appetite loss	stress	spasms

other _____

product used _____

dosage _____

method _____

other meds _____

NOTES

Did your symptoms improve, stay the same, or get worse?

DATE

SYMPTOMS

cramping	muscle pain	seizures
anxiety	nerve pain	headache
fatigue	joint pain	dizziness
depression	nausea	eye pressure
appetite loss	stress	spasms

other _____

product used _____

dosage _____

method _____

other meds _____

NOTES

Did your symptoms improve, stay the same, or get worse?

DATE

SYMPTOMS

cramping	muscle pain	seizures
anxiety	nerve pain	headache
fatigue	joint pain	dizziness
depression	nausea	eye pressure
appetite loss	stress	spasms

other _____

product used _____

dosage _____

method _____

other meds _____

NOTES

Did your symptoms improve, stay the same, or get worse?

DATE

SYMPTOMS

cramping	muscle pain	seizures
anxiety	nerve pain	headache
fatigue	joint pain	dizziness
depression	nausea	eye pressure
appetite loss	stress	spasms

other _____

product used _____

dosage _____

method _____

other meds _____

NOTES

Did your symptoms improve, stay the same, or get worse?

DATE

SYMPTOMS

cramping	muscle pain	seizures
anxiety	nerve pain	headache
fatigue	joint pain	dizziness
depression	nausea	eye pressure
appetite loss	stress	spasms

other _____

product used _____

dosage _____

method _____

other meds _____

NOTES

Did your symptoms improve, stay the same, or get worse?

DATE

SYMPTOMS

cramping	muscle pain	seizures
anxiety	nerve pain	headache
fatigue	joint pain	dizziness
depression	nausea	eye pressure
appetite loss	stress	spasms

other _____

product used _____

dosage _____

method _____

other meds _____

NOTES

Did your symptoms improve, stay the same, or get worse?

DATE

SYMPTOMS

cramping	muscle pain	seizures
anxiety	nerve pain	headache
fatigue	joint pain	dizziness
depression	nausea	eye pressure
appetite loss	stress	spasms

other _____

product used _____

dosage _____

method _____

other meds _____

NOTES

Did your symptoms improve, stay the same, or get worse?

DATE

SYMPTOMS

cramping	muscle pain	seizures
anxiety	nerve pain	headache
fatigue	joint pain	dizziness
depression	nausea	eye pressure
appetite loss	stress	spasms

other _____

product used _____

dosage _____

method _____

other meds _____

NOTES

Did your symptoms improve, stay the same, or get worse?

DATE

SYMPTOMS

cramping	muscle pain	seizures
anxiety	nerve pain	headache
fatigue	joint pain	dizziness
depression	nausea	eye pressure
appetite loss	stress	spasms

other _____

product used _____

dosage _____

method _____

other meds _____

NOTES

Did your symptoms improve, stay the same, or get worse?

DATE

SYMPTOMS

cramping	muscle pain	seizures
anxiety	nerve pain	headache
fatigue	joint pain	dizziness
depression	nausea	eye pressure
appetite loss	stress	spasms

other _____

product used _____

dosage _____

method _____

other meds _____

NOTES

Did your symptoms improve, stay the same, or get worse?

DATE

SYMPTOMS

cramping	muscle pain	seizures
anxiety	nerve pain	headache
fatigue	joint pain	dizziness
depression	nausea	eye pressure
appetite loss	stress	spasms
	other _____	

product used _____

dosage _____

method _____

other meds _____

NOTES

Did your symptoms improve, stay the same, or get worse?

DATE

SYMPTOMS

cramping	muscle pain	seizures
anxiety	nerve pain	headache
fatigue	joint pain	dizziness
depression	nausea	eye pressure
appetite loss	stress	spasms

other _____

product used _____

dosage _____

method _____

other meds _____

NOTES

Did your symptoms improve, stay the same, or get worse?

DATE

SYMPTOMS

cramping	muscle pain	seizures
anxiety	nerve pain	headache
fatigue	joint pain	dizziness
depression	nausea	eye pressure
appetite loss	stress	spasms

other _____

product used _____

dosage _____

method _____

other meds _____

NOTES

Did your symptoms improve, stay the same, or get worse?

DATE

SYMPTOMS

cramping muscle pain seizures

anxiety nerve pain headache

fatigue joint pain dizziness

depression nausea eye pressure

appetite loss stress spasms

other _____

product used _____

dosage _____

method _____

other meds _____

NOTES

Did your symptoms improve, stay the same, or get worse?

DATE

SYMPTOMS

cramping	muscle pain	seizures
anxiety	nerve pain	headache
fatigue	joint pain	dizziness
depression	nausea	eye pressure
appetite loss	stress	spasms

other _____

product used _____

dosage _____

method _____

other meds _____

NOTES

Did your symptoms improve, stay the same, or get worse?

DATE

SYMPTOMS

cramping	muscle pain	seizures
anxiety	nerve pain	headache
fatigue	joint pain	dizziness
depression	nausea	eye pressure
appetite loss	stress	spasms

other _____

product used _____

dosage _____

method _____

other meds _____

NOTES

Did your symptoms improve, stay the same, or get worse?

DATE

SYMPTOMS

cramping	muscle pain	seizures
anxiety	nerve pain	headache
fatigue	joint pain	dizziness
depression	nausea	eye pressure
appetite loss	stress	spasms

other _____

product used _____

dosage _____

method _____

other meds _____

NOTES

Did your symptoms improve, stay the same, or get worse?

DATE

SYMPTOMS

cramping	muscle pain	seizures
anxiety	nerve pain	headache
fatigue	joint pain	dizziness
depression	nausea	eye pressure
appetite loss	stress	spasms

other _____

product used _____

dosage _____

method _____

other meds _____

NOTES

Did your symptoms improve, stay the same, or get worse?